LINDA PARKER

Gentle Movement: Low-Impact Exercises for Seniors with Joint Pain

A Guide to Joint-Friendly Exercises To Help Gain Balance, Stability, Flexibility, and Strength

This book was professionally typeset on Reedsy.
Find out more at reedsy.com

Contents

1

Introduction

Welcome to a journey of renewal and empowerment, a guide designed to help enrich the lives of seniors struggling with the challenges of joint pain. As you turn these pages, you're not just reading a book; you're opening the door to a world where age is not a barrier but a pathway to rediscovering the joy of movement and your body's resilience.

For many of us, aging accompanies the unwelcome companions of stiffness and discomfort. Joint pain, a common ailment in our later years, can feel like an anchor, weighing down our bodies and spirits. However, it's crucial to recognize that movement is not the enemy; our inaction is. My goal in writing this book was to be your ally and provide you with a guide in breaking free from the cycle of pain and inactivity.

The importance of staying active as we age cannot be overstated. Physical activity, especially exercises tailored for seniors, is pivotal in maintaining and enhancing our quality of life. It's about more than just keeping fit; it's about sustaining our independence, nurturing our mental health, and cherishing our connections with ourselves and the world around us. Yet, the key is finding the right types of exercise.

Activities gentle enough for our joints yet effective in keeping us agile, lively, and in the game!

Low-impact exercises are the heart of this journey. These activities are our tools to enhance mobility, reduce pain, and rekindle the energy of youth. They are carefully designed to be gentle yet effective, ensuring the path to fitness is safe, enjoyable, and rewarding. Whether it's gaining balance and stability, enhancing flexibility, or building strength, these exercises are tailored to suit our unique needs and capabilities.

However, before we embark on this journey together, caution is essential. Each body is unique, and what works for one may not work for another. Therefore, consulting with medical professionals before starting any new exercise regimen is important. This step is not just a formality; it's a cornerstone of responsible self-care. Your healthcare provider can offer invaluable insights into how these exercises can best be adapted to your health profile, ensuring that your path to wellness is effective and safe.

As we move forward, remember that this book is more than just a collection of exercises. It's a celebration of your determination, a testament to your resilience, and a tribute to your desire to live every moment with vitality and joy. So, let's get moving on this journey together, embracing each day with a renewed sense of purpose and the knowledge that our best years can indeed lie ahead of us. Welcome to your new chapter of fitness and vitality.

2

Understanding Joint Pain in Seniors

Understanding the medical causes of joint pain in seniors sets a solid foundation for adopting appropriate low-impact exercises. Recognizing the role of aging in joint health helps adopt a proactive approach to maintain mobility and quality of life, debunking the myth that aging inevitably confines one to a sedentary lifestyle. This chapter aims to empower you with knowledge, paving the way for a more active, pain-managed, and fulfilling senior life.

As we age, our bodies undergo inevitable changes. Our joints, the connectors between bones, are particularly susceptible. They wear down over time, primarily due to the breakdown of cartilage – the protective cushioning inside joints. This process, known as osteoarthritis, is the most common cause of joint pain among seniors. A simplified explanation is that synovial fluid, which acts as a lubricant, decreases, increasing friction and pain in our joints during movement.

Another medical cause is rheumatoid arthritis, an autoimmune disorder where the body's immune system mistakenly attacks the joints, causing inflammation and pain. Other conditions like gout, bursitis, and tendinitis also contribute to joint pain, emphasizing the variety of triggers seniors might experience. Muscle strength also diminishes with age, putting additional strain on joints. Without adequate muscle support, joints become more susceptible to injury and inflammation, compounding pain. These are only a few conditions that may cause joint pain; please consult your physician to determine if your aches and pains are caused by aging or another underlying condition.

Contrary to the myth that exercise worsens joint pain, physical activity is not just safe but essential. Regular, low-impact exercise helps maintain joint flexibility, reduces pain, and slows the progression of joint-related diseases. It improves blood flow, delivers nutrients to joint tissues, and helps remove waste products.

Joint pain, a frequent companion in our senior years, often becomes a significant barrier to an active and enjoyable life. Understanding its causes and effects is the first step in managing this condition effectively and embracing a lifestyle that accommodates, rather than aggravates, this common ailment. There is so much more, and we could look deeper into all the causes of joint pain, but I'll leave any further discussions between you and your healthcare provider.

3

The Principles of Low-Impact Exercises

In fitness, especially for those over 60 facing joint pain, understanding, and adopting low-impact exercises is not just beneficial; it is essential. This chapter delves into the fundamentals of low-impact exercise, shedding light on its nature, its significance for seniors, and how it distinctly differs from high-impact activities.

What is Low-Impact Exercise?

Low-impact exercise refers to activities where at least one foot always remains in contact with the ground, or the body is not jumping, slamming, or bumping – no jarring movements. This definition is crucial as it highlights the gentle nature of these exercises on the joints. They are designed to impose minimal stress on the body's weight-bearing joints, including the hips, knees, and ankles. Examples include walking, cycling, swimming, yoga, and several forms of dance.

The primary appeal of low-impact exercise lies in its accessibility and adaptability. It is particularly beneficial for individuals who are older or recovering from injuries, as well as those with chronic conditions such as arthritis or osteoporosis. However, its benefits are not limited to these groups alone; low-impact workouts can be an effective part of anyone's fitness regime, offering cardiovascular, strength, and endurance training without the harsh impact of more intense exercises.

Why Low-Impact for Seniors?

Low-impact exercise is particularly beneficial for seniors, offering a safe and effective way to maintain physical health and enhance quality of life without putting undue strain on the body. As we age, our bodies naturally change - decreased bone density, reduced muscle mass, and the increased likelihood of joint-related issues, which is the primary focus of this book. Low-impact exercises minimize stress on joints, bones, and muscles by their gentle nature, reducing the risk of injury and pain that can come from more high-impact activities.

Maintaining mobility and independence is crucial for seniors, and low-impact exercises such as walking, swimming, yoga, and tai chi can significantly contribute to this goal. Incorporating low-impact exercises into a senior's routine can lead to a more active, healthier lifestyle, increasing longevity and a better quality of life in later years.

The Contrast with High-Impact Activities

High-impact exercises involve activities where both feet leave the ground simultaneously, even momentarily. These exercises are characterized by greater force or impact exerted on the body, especially on the weight-bearing joints such as the knees, hips, and ankles, such as running, jumping, or certain aerobic workouts. While beneficial for younger individuals or those without joint issues, they can be detrimental for seniors, especially those with arthritis or pre-existing joint pain, due to the increased stress on the joints.

Tips Approaching Low-Impact Exercises Safely

1. **Consult a medical professional**: As stated several times, please speak with your physician before starting any new physical activity program. Once in the clear, go for it!

2. **Start with a Warm-Up:** Beginning any exercise routine with a warm-up is crucial. It prepares the body for physical activity by increasing blood flow to the muscles, thus reducing the risk of injury. Simple, light stretching or a brisk five to ten-minute walk can suffice. This is not where you want to overdo it. You are looking to warm your body up for the main activity.

3. **Understand Your Limits:** Recognizing and respecting your body's limits is key. If you experience pain beyond the usual "workout burn," it's a signal to stop. Pushing through pain can lead to injury. The goal is to use low-impact exercises to improve your stability, balance, flexibility, and strength, not cause injury.

4. **Consistency Over Intensity:** For seniors, regular exercise is more important than intensity. Consistent, moderate exercise is more beneficial than sporadic, intense workouts. Plan a weekly exercise routine and schedule days for different activities. And low-impact exercise is great for all age levels, so find family and friends to exercise with you!

5. **Balance Your Routine:** A well-rounded exercise routine should include cardiovascular training, strength building, flexibility, and stability/balance training. This approach ensures all areas of fitness are covered. Remember to mix up the training when you are planning your weekly exercises.

6. **Stay Hydrated and Nourished:** Proper hydration and nutrition

are essential. You should drink water before, during, and after exercise and follow a balanced diet to fuel your body. Investing in a refillable water bottle is like investing in yourself! It doesn't have to be fancy but should hold enough water to get you through the day.

7. **Use Proper Equipment:** Using the right equipment, such as supportive footwear, can significantly reduce the risk of injury. Consider getting fitted for proper footwear if you experience issues such as plantar fasciitis or need arch supports. In the case of exercises like cycling or swimming, ensuring the equipment is properly adjusted and maintained is important. If you are completing your exercises in a public gym, wipe down any equipment you may use before and after use. If you are outside, watch out for cracks in sidewalks or uneven pavements.

8. **Cool Down:** Conclude each exercise session with a cool-down period. Gentle stretching for 5-10 minutes helps the body transition back to a resting state and can reduce muscle stiffness. Don't forget to hydrate!

Understanding Modifications and Adaptations

Adaptation is key in low-impact exercises. If an exercise causes discomfort, modifying it to a less intense version or using aids like chairs for balance can be helpful. Consulting a physical therapist or a trained instructor for personalized modifications can be highly beneficial. In the next chapter, I will also discuss exercise equipment modifications.There is no excuse for not finding one or several low-impact exercises to fit into a routine.

Monitoring Progress and Adjusting Routines

Keep track of your exercise routine and its effects on your body. If certain activities become easier, it may be time to increase the intensity or duration slightly. Conversely, scaling back or modifying activities is necessary if they become difficult or painful. Remember, what works for one person may not work for someone else. The key is finding the right low-impact exercises to fit your needs.

The Role of Technology in Low-Impact Exercises

In this digital age, seniors (and almost everyone) can access many resources online, from exercise tutorials to virtual classes, making it easier to find suitable low-impact exercises and follow along from the comfort of their homes. If you feel you are not tech-savvy enough to access technology, there are resources in many communities that can assist with getting you set up. Also, consider contacting your local high school or community college to inquire about students studying information technology and looking for a side job setting up streaming services for you. There is technology help out there!

A final thought…low-impact exercises are a cornerstone of maintaining health and mobility in seniors, particularly those with joint pain. By understanding and applying the principles outlined in this chapter, seniors can safely and effectively engage in physical activities, enhancing their overall well-being. Remember, the goal is not to overdo it but to find the right level of low-impact exercise that will provide an effective outcome for you. See you in Chapter 3 for the low-impact exercises!

4

Essential Low-Impact Exercises

This core chapter provides descriptions, benefits, step-by-step guides, and resources for 20 low-impact exercises designed for seniors experiencing joint issues. Each exercise is designed to be gentle on the joints while gaining balance and stability, enhancing flexibility, building strength, and enhancing cardiovascular health as a bonus! This is the heart of the guidebook and what I hope will help you create a low-impact routine that will work for you.

Stretching: Gentle stretches to improve flexibility.

Benefits: Increases flexibility and reduces muscle tension.

Steps: Include stretches for all major muscle groups, holding each stretch for 15-30 seconds. Modify stretching routines by sitting in a chair. Here are some common stretching routines to get you started:

- Overhead side stretching routine: standing tall with legs hip-width apart, raising arms over your head. Interlocking your fingers is optional. Lean gently to one side and hold for 15-30 seconds; return to the center, then lean to the other side.

- Hamstring stretching routine: place one of your heels on a low bench with your leg straight and toes pointed up. Gently lower lean forward bending at the hip while keeping your lower back straight until you feel a comfortable stretch.Hold for 15-30 seconds, release, switch legs, and repeat.
- Calf stretching routine: you can perform this stretch near a wall or chair for balance. Stand with one leg in front of you slightly bent and your opposite leg straight behind you. Press the heel of the back straight leg into the floor to feel a comfortable stretch, hold for 15-30 seconds, release, switch legs, and repeat.

Walking: It's probably not surprising to many that walking is near the top of the list. It requires little investment other than a great pair of walking shoes and can be easily modified for ability. It's a simple, effective aerobic exercise that enhances cardiovascular health.

Benefits: Improves heart health, strengthens leg muscles, and boosts mood.

Steps: Start with a comfortable pace, gradually increasing duration and speed. Aim for 30 minutes a day. Reminder: stay hydrated!

Resources: Don't let bad weather stop you! Have a smartphone? There are apps available that will take you through guided indoor walking routines.

Yoga: Gentle, flexible exercise enhancing mind-body connection and stress relief.

Benefits: Improves flexibility and balance, reduces joint pain, promotes mental well-being, and increases strength.

Steps: Tabletop Pose (Bharmanasana) in yoga involves a simple yet effective position that forms the foundation for many other poses. It's a great pose for building strength in the spine and torso, improving posture, and creating body awareness. Always listen to your body and adjust as needed for comfort and safety.

- Begin by kneeling on a yoga mat or a comfortable surface. Position your knees directly under your hips and your wrists under your shoulders. Your shins and knees should be hip-width apart.
- Keep your back flat, like a tabletop, and your neck a natural extension of your spine. Avoid arching your back or letting your belly sag.
- Look down at the mat, aligning your head with your spine. This position will help maintain a neutral neck and avoid any strain.
- Spread your fingers wide and press through the base of each finger. This helps in distributing your weight evenly and reduces pressure on your wrists.
- Activate your abdominal muscles to support your spine. This engagement is subtle but crucial for maintaining a stable and aligned posture.
- Hold this position, breathing steadily. Ensure that your shoulders are away from your ears, creating space in the neck area.
- Modification: If you have knee discomfort, use a folded blanket or a knee pad for extra cushioning. If you feel wrist strain, make fists with your hands or use yoga blocks under your palms to alleviate pressure. Focus on keeping your hips and shoulders square and aligned with each other.

Steps: Cat-Cow Pose (Marjaryasana-Bitilasana) – a great pose that combines a flow between two poses. This pose will warm your body, improve your posture and flexibility, and increase your blood flow.

- Start on your hands and knees in a tabletop (beginning position), with your wrists directly under your shoulders and your knees under your hips.

- As you inhale, arch your back, dropping your belly towards the mat, and lift your head and tailbone upward (Cow Pose).
- As you exhale, round your back towards the ceiling, tucking your chin towards your chest and bringing your tailbone down (Cat Pose).
- Continue flowing between these two poses for several breaths, moving with your breath rhythm.

Steps: Mountain Pose (Tadasana) – a good beginning pose that helps correct muscle imbalance and improve posture and alignment. Caution: If you suffer from high or low blood pressure or are prone to migraines, leave this pose to others since holding the position for too long could lead to dizziness.

- Stand with your feet together or hip-width apart, spreading your toes wide and grounding through your feet.
- Engage your thighs to lift your kneecaps slightly, keeping a slight bend in the knees to avoid locking them.
- Lengthen your spine, roll your shoulders back and down, and let your arms hang naturally with palms facing forward.
- Hold the pose for several breaths, focusing on standing tall and steady.

Chair Yoga: Yoga poses modified for sitting in a chair.

Benefits: Enhances flexibility, reduces stress, and improves joint mobility. Include gentle stretches and breathing exercises. Focus on flexibility and balance.

Steps: Chair Mountain Pose (Tadasana)

- Sit upright at the edge of a chair with your feet flat on the ground.
- Keep your back straight and your hands resting on your thighs or lifted above your head.
- Engage your leg muscles and core as if standing.

Steps: Chair Cat-Cow Stretch:

- Sit on a chair with your feet flat on the ground and spine straight.
- Place your hands on your knees.
- Inhale, arch your back, and look up towards the ceiling (Cow).
- Exhale, round your spine, and tuck your chin to your chest (Cat).
- Continue flowing between these two poses.

Water Aerobics: Cardio and strength exercises performed in a pool.

Benefits: Lowers impact on joints, improves endurance, and builds strength.

Steps: Attend guided classes for structured routines. Include movements like leg kicks and arm sweeps.

Resources: Many communities have local senior centers or community center swimming pools that offer water aerobics or swimming hours. Take advantage of any local resources or neighbors if you do not have a swimming pool.

Tai Chi: a gentle form of martial arts that focuses on slow, deliberate movements.

Benefits: Improves balance, reduces stress, and aids in joint health.

Steps: Begin with basic forms, gradually learning sequences. Practice regularly. Here are a few forms suitable for beginners, but online lessons are available.

Opening and Closing Hands:

- Stand with your feet shoulder-width apart and knees slightly bent.
- Relax your shoulders and gently rest your hands at your sides.
- Slowly raise your arms before you, palms facing down while inhaling.
- Turn your palms up and gently draw your hands towards your chest as if gathering energy, then push your palms outward while exhaling.
- Repeat this open-and-close movement several times, focusing on the flow of your breath with your movements.

Wave Hands Like Clouds:

- Stand with your feet a comfortable distance apart.
- Raise your arms to chest height and gently sway them from side to side as if moving them through clouds.
- Keep your wrists relaxed and your movements fluid.
- Your gaze follows your moving hand, and your waist guides the movement.

Stationary Cycling: Cycling on a stationary bike.

Benefits: Strengthens leg muscles, improves joint mobility, and boosts cardiovascular health.

Steps: Start with a light resistance, gradually increasing as comfort grows. Aim for 30 minutes a day.

Resources: exercise equipment comes in a wide cost range, but you don't have to break the bank looking for a stationary bike. Social media marketplaces are a great place to find exercise equipment, often nearly new. Also, using a recumbent bike is a great modification to this activity if you feel you have balance issues.

Pilates: A low-impact exercise that emphasizes body alignment and core strength.

Benefits: Enhances core strength, improves posture, and increases flexibility.

Steps: Focus on controlled movements and breathing. Start with beginner exercises.

Resources: Many health organizations have weighed in on the overwhelming benefits of Pilates for seniors. There are in-person, virtual, and recorded classes; you name it, Pilates is everywhere! I caution you to find a qualified instructor, read reviews of local instructors, ask for recommendations, and discuss physical limitations with your instructor.

Leg Lifts: Simple strengthening exercise targeting the legs and lower abdomen.

Benefits: Strengthens legs and abdominal muscles and improves balance.

Steps: Lie on your back and lift one leg at a time. Keep movements slow and controlled. Here is an alternative to the standard leg lift exercise.

Seated Knee Lifts (Strengthens thighs and improves joint mobility)

- Sit in a sturdy chair with your feet flat on the ground.
- Slowly lift one knee towards your chest as comfortably as possible.
- Lower it back down with control.
- Alternate legs, doing 10-15 lifts per leg.

Arm Raises: Strengthens shoulders and arms using light weights or resistance bands.

Benefits: Builds upper body strength and improves joint flexibility.

Steps: Can be modified for standing or seated; no weights, weights, or resistance bands.

Front Arm Raises (Targets the front shoulders)

- Stand or sit with your back straight and arms at your sides.
- Slowly lift your arms straight in front of you to shoulder height, palms facing down.
- Lower them back down with control.
- Perform 10-15 repetitions.

Lateral Arm Raises (Works on the side shoulders)

- Start in the same initial position as the front arm raises.
- Raise your arms to the sides, keeping them straight, up to shoulder height.
- Slowly lower them back to your sides.
- Do 10-15 repetitions.

Presses (Strengthens the entire shoulder)

- Sit or stand with your arms bent, elbows at shoulder height, and palms facing forward.
- Extend your arms straight above your head.
- Bring them back to shoulder height.
- Complete 10-15 repetitions.

Seated Rowing: A rowing motion performed while sitting, using a resistance band.

Benefits: Strengthens back and arms, improves posture.

Steps: Pull the band towards your waist while seated, keeping your back straight.

Resources: This is a great alternative if you cannot access a rowing machine. However, if you are interested in this type of activity, check out local social media marketplaces and you might find a deal on a rowing machine.

Step-Ups: Stepping onto a low platform and back down.

Benefits: Builds leg strength and enhances coordination.

Steps: Use a sturdy, low step. Step up with one foot, then the other, and reverse. Hold onto a chair for balance if necessary.

Heel-to-Toe Walk: Improves balance and lower body strength.

Benefits: Improves balance and gait, strengthens lower body.

Steps: Walk in a straight line, placing your heel directly in front of the toe of the opposite foot. Complete this exercise next to a wall or barre if you need assistance with balance.

Wall Push-Ups: A modified push-up against a wall.

Benefits: Strengthens chest and arms, lessens strain on back and shoulders.

Steps: Face a wall with your feet hip-width apart for stability. Place your palms flat against the wall at shoulder height and width apart, fingers pointing upwards. Take a small step back so your feet are not directly under your shoulders, creating a slight angle in your body. Ensure your body is straight from your head to your heels. Inhale as you slowly bend your elbows and bring your chest towards the wall. Keep your elbows pointing downwards, not flaring out to the sides. Go as close to the wall as you can while maintaining good form. Exhale as you push yourself back to the starting position by straightening your arms. Make sure to keep your body straight and rigid throughout the movement. Perform the desired number of repetitions. Start with a number that feels comfortable, typically, 10 to 15 push-ups are a good starting point.

Bicep Curls: Using light weights to strengthen arm muscles. You can perform bicep curls either standing or sitting. If standing, ensure your feet are hip-width apart for stability. If sitting, choose a chair without arms to allow free movement of your arms.

Benefits: Increases upper body strength and improves joint mobility.

Steps: Hold a weight in each hand with your arms hanging down at your sides. Ensure your palms are facing forward. Keep your elbows close to your torso and your spine straight. Exhale and slowly curl the weights up towards your shoulders by bending your elbows and contracting your biceps. Keep your upper arms stationary. Pause momentarily once your biceps are fully contracted and the weights are at shoulder level. Inhale as you slowly lower the weights back to the starting position. Maintain control and do not let the weights drop; the downward movement is as important as the curl-up. Perform 8-12 repetitions, depending on your comfort and fitness level.

Ankle Circles: Rotating the ankles to improve mobility and reduce stiffness.

Benefits: Enhances ankle flexibility, reduces stiffness.

Steps: You can perform ankle circles while sitting or lying down. If sitting, choose a chair where you can comfortably sit with your feet not touching the ground. Extend one leg out in front of you. If lying down, you can keep the other leg flat on the surface, and if sitting, let it hang naturally. Begin rotating your ankle, moving only your ankle and foot, keeping your leg still. Rotate your ankle in a circular motion, making as large a circle as is comfortable. After doing 10-15 circles in one direction, reverse and rotate your ankle in the opposite direction for an equal number of circles. After completing the rotations on one ankle, switch to the other leg and repeat the exercise.

Seated Toe Taps: A simple leg exercise that can be done while sitting.

Benefits: Improves leg strength, enhances circulation.

Steps: Sit in a sturdy, stable chair. Your feet should rest flat on the floor with knees bent at about a 90-degree angle. Ensure the chair doesn't have wheels for safety. Sit up straight with your back against the chair's backrest. Your shoulders should be relaxed, and your hands can rest on your thighs or the arms of the chair. With both feet flat on the floor, hip-width apart, lift the toes of one foot as high as you comfortably can while keeping your heel on the ground. You should feel the muscles in your shin working. Tap your toes back down to the floor in a gentle, controlled movement. Continue this up-and-down tapping motion. After completing a set of repetitions with one foot, switch to the other foot and repeat the exercise. Aim to perform about 10-15 toe taps per foot to start. As you build strength and flexibility, you can increase the number of repetitions.

Balancing Exercises: Exercises to improve balance and stability.

Benefits: Improves balance, reduces risk of falls.

Steps: Practices like standing on one foot or side-stepping.

Standing on one foot:

- Stand behind a chair and hold onto it for support.
- Lift one foot a few inches off the ground, balancing on the other foot.
- Hold the position for as long as you can, then switch feet.
- Aim for 10-30 seconds on each leg.

Side-Stepping:

- Stand with your feet together and a chair in front for support.
- Step to the side in a slow and controlled manner, then step back to the starting position.
- Do 10-15 steps on each side.

Shoulder Shrugs: Lifting and lowering shoulders to relieve tension and build strength. This exercise can be performed seated.

Benefits: Reduces neck and shoulder tension, increases strength.

Steps: Stand or sit upright with your feet hip-width apart. If standing, ensure your knees have a slight bend to avoid locking them. Let your arms hang naturally at your sides with your palms facing your body. Inhale and lift your shoulders towards your ears as high as you comfortably can. Try to make the movement smooth and controlled. Keep your neck straight and your arms relaxed, the movement should be in your shoulders only. Hold the shrug for a moment at the top of the movement to maximize the stretch in your shoulders and neck. Exhale and slowly lower your shoulders back to the starting position. Repeat the shrugs for 10-15 repetitions, or as many as feel comfortable.

Seated Marching: Mimicking a marching motion while seated.

Benefits: Strengthens legs, improves flexibility, enhances circulation.

Steps: Sit in a sturdy chair that allows your feet to touch the ground while keeping your knees at a 90-degree angle. Chairs with no arms are best for this activity. Sit up straight with your back against the chair. Place your feet flat on the floor, hip-width apart. Lift your right knee towards your chest as high as comfortably possible. Lower your right foot back to the floor. Then lift your left knee towards your chest. Continue alternating legs, mimicking a marching motion. As you march, engage your core muscles to maintain your posture. You can swing your arms in opposition to your legs for more engagement. Make your movements controlled and deliberate. Focus on lifting your knees as high as you comfortably can. Breathe evenly throughout the exercise. Inhale as you lift your knee and exhale as you lower it. Start with a short duration, like 1-2 minutes, and gradually increase as your endurance improves.

Each exercise is designed to be gentle on the joints while effectively strengthening muscles, improving flexibility, and enhancing cardiovascular health. Always remember to listen to your body and consult with medical professionals to tailor these exercises to your specific needs. Remember, the goal is to maintain and improve your quality of life, making every movement count towards a healthier, more vibrant you.

5

Creating Your Personal Low-Impact Exercise Routine

Before beginning any new exercise program, especially if you have joint pain or other health issues, it's crucial to consult with your medical professional. They can provide personalized advice ensuring the exercises are safe and beneficial for your specific condition. Here is my weekly routine and additional sample exercise routines to get you started.They are designed from the low-impact exercises discussed in the previous chapter, and you can use them as they are or modify them to fit your schedule, the combinations are limitless.

Linda's Routine:

Day 1: Walking and Stretching

Morning: 30-minute walk at a comfortable pace.

Evening: 20 minutes of stretching, emphasizing areas that feel particularly tight/sore.

Nighttime: 12 minutes of meditation

Day 2: Strength Training and Recumbent Bicycle

Morning: 20 minutes of light strength training using light weights.

Evening: 30 minutes on recumbent bike

Nighttime: 12 minutes of meditation

Day 3: Pilates and Stretching:

Morning: 20 minutes of gentle Pilates for beginners (streaming service)

Evening: 20 minutes of stretching, emphasizing areas that feel particularly tight/sore.

Nighttime: 12 minutes of meditation

Day 4: Rest Day

Morning: I usually do a light stretch and morning meditation.

Nighttime: 20 minute meditation

Day 5: Walking and Chair Exercises

Morning: 30-minute walk at a comfortable pace.

Evening: 20 minutes of seated exercises, including arm raises and bicep curls.

Nighttime: 12 minutes of meditation

Day 6: Recumbent Bicycle and Stretching

Morning: 30 minutes on recumbent bike

Evening: 20 minutes of stretching, emphasizing areas that feel particularly tight/sore.

Nighttime: 12 minutes of meditation

Day 7: Gentle Yoga and Balance/Flexibility

Morning: 20 minutes of gentle yoga focusing on slow movements and deep breathing.

Evening: 15 minutes of stretching or a relaxing yoga session to enhance flexibility.

Nighttime: 12 minutes of meditation

Sample Routine 1:

Day 1: Gentle Yoga and Stretching

Morning: 20 minutes of gentle yoga focusing on slow movements and deep breathing.

Evening: 15 minutes of stretching, emphasizing areas that feel particularly tight/sore.

Day 2: Water Aerobics

Morning/Afternoon: Attend a 30-minute water aerobics class, which is excellent

for joint pain due to the low-impact nature of water exercises.

Day 3: Walking and Balance Exercises

Morning: 20-minute walk at a comfortable pace.

Evening: 10 minutes of balancing exercises such as standing on one leg

or side-stepping.

Day 4: Rest Day

Use this day to rest and recover. Engage in light activities like casual walking

or some gentle stretching if you feel up to it.

Day 5: Chair Exercises

Morning: 20 minutes of seated exercises, including seated marching, leg lifts,

and arm raises.

Evening: 15 minutes of gentle stretching or yoga poses suitable for doing in a chair.

Day 6: Tai Chi

Morning: Join a 30-minute Tai Chi class, ideal for improving balance and

reducing stress, while being gentle on the joints.

Day 7: Strength Training

Morning: 20 minutes of light strength training using light weights or resistance bands. Focus on exercises like bicep curls or shoulder shrugs.

Evening: End the week with 15 minutes of stretching or a relaxing yoga

session to enhance flexibility.

Sample Routine 2:

Day 1: Walking and Gentle Stretching

Morning: Start with a 20-minute walk at a comfortable, steady pace.

Evening: Spend 15 minutes doing gentle stretching exercises, focusing on areas

that feel tight or sore.

Day 2: Pilates Basics

Morning: Engage in a 30-minute beginner Pilates session, focusing on

core strength and stability.

Evening: Cool down with 10 minutes of deep breathing exercises.

Day 3: Balance and Flexibility

Morning: Perform balance exercises like side-stepping or single-leg stands
for 15 minutes.
Evening: 20 minutes of yoga focusing on poses that enhance flexibility and balance.

Day 4: Rest Day

Allow your body to rest and recover. Engage in light activities such as casual walking
or gentle stretching if you feel up to it.

Day 5: Chair Exercises

Morning: 25 minutes of seated exercises, including seated leg lifts, arm raises,
and gentle upper body twists.
Evening: 15 minutes of relaxation and breathing exercises.

Day 6: Walking and Light Strength Training

Morning: Take a 25-minute walk, possibly including some slight inclines for
a bit more challenge.
Evening: 20 minutes of light strength training using resistance bands or
light dumbbells for upper body exercises like bicep curls or shoulder presses.

Day 7: Tai Chi and Stretching

Morning: Participate in a 30-minute Tai Chi session, focusing on gentle,
flowing movements.
Evening: Wrap up the week with a 20-minute stretching session,

focusing on
    full-body relaxation and flexibility.

No excuses, start by finding a good time of day to workout. Be consistent and then add on as you get stronger!

6

Beyond Exercise - Holistic Approaches to Managing Joint Pain in Seniors

Joint pain in seniors is a prevalent issue that can significantly impact the quality of life. A holistic approach to managing this pain focuses on treating the whole person, considering physical, emotional, and environmental factors, rather than just the symptoms. So far, we have focused primarily on exercise and physical activity and to a lesser degree the mind-body connection with the practice of yoga and tai chi. I want to discuss some other holistic strategies that can be effective in managing joint pain in older adults.

Mind-Body Practices: Yoga and tai chi were outlined as low-impact exercises, but an additional form of mind-body practice that I have found incredibly beneficial as a personal strategy is meditation. Along with yoga and tai chi, mediation helps in stress reduction, which is important as stress can intensify pain perception. There are a lot of different guided meditation platforms popping up, but I am a huge fan of the Calm app on my smartphone. There is guided meditation, sleep stories, music, and so much more.If you are looking to develop mindfulness, it's a good place to start.

Diet and Nutrition: A balanced diet plays a crucial role in managing joint pain. Foods rich in omega-3 fatty acids, such as salmon and flaxseeds, can reduce inflammation. Incorporating fruits and vegetables, high in antioxidants, helps combat oxidative stress that can exacerbate joint pain. Seniors should also stay hydrated and consider adding supplements like glucosamine and chondroitin after consulting with a healthcare provider.

Here's a great recipe for GRILLED SALMON AND LEMON ASPARAGUS FOIL PACKS. Recipe will work with any kind of seafood or vegetable. It's super easy and serves 4.

INGREDIENTS:
  16-20 asparagus spears (or seasonal vegetable)
  4 – 6 oz, skin on salmon filets (wild-caught is best)
  4 tablespoons butter, divided
  2 lemons, sliced
  Kosher salt
  Ground black pepper
  Fresh parsley or dill, for garnish (optional)

COOKING DIRECTIONS:

Lay four pieces of foil on a flat surface. Place 4-5 spears of asparagus on foil and top with a filet of salmon, 1 tablespoon of butter, two slices of lemon, salt and pepper to taste. Loosely wrap, then repeat with remaining ingredients until you have four packets total.

Heat grill on high.Add foil packets to grill and cook until salmon is cooked through, and asparagus is tender, about 10 minutes. Garnish and serve…it's that simple!

Complementary Therapies: Acupuncture and massage therapy can be effective in pain management. Acupuncture stimulates specific points of the body to balance energy flow, while massage helps in reducing muscle tension and improving circulation. Both therapies can improve joint mobility and function. Acupuncture can help in restoring balance and promoting the body's natural healing processes, leading to better joint movement. Massage therapy, through various techniques, can increase flexibility, reduce stiffness, and improve range of motion in the joints.

Lifestyle Modifications: Adding low-impact movement, hydration, and maintaining a balanced diet have all been discussed but there are other modifications we can make to improve the quality of our lives.Adequate sleep and stress management are crucial. Good sleep allows for the healing and repair of cells and tissues, while poor sleep can intensify pain sensitivity and overall discomfort. Chronic stress can worsen pain perception. Techniques such as deep breathing, meditation, and mindfulness can help in reducing stress and its impact on joint pain. Creating an ergonomic living space can also help in reducing strain on joints during daily activities.

Herbal Remedies: Certain herbs like turmeric, ginger, and green tea have anti-inflammatory properties that can alleviate joint pain. However, it's important to discuss with a healthcare provider before starting any herbal remedies, especially for seniors with existing health conditions or those on medication. Personally, I am a green tea fiend. I start my day with dandelion green tea and end with peppermint green tea.

Community and Emotional Support: Joining support groups or engaging in community activities can provide emotional support and reduce feelings of isolation, which can positively impact overall well-being. The Centers for Disease and Control and Prevention has a community program called Fit & Strong!, check it out on their website to see if it's right for you. https://www.cdc.gov/arthritis/interventions/programs/fit-strong.htm

A holistic approach to managing joint pain in seniors involves a combination of dietary choices, physical activity, mind-body practices, complementary therapies, lifestyle changes, and emotional support. It's vital to consult healthcare professionals to customize these strategies to individual needs and conditions.

7

Conclusion

The low-impact exercises introduced in this book are by no means all-inclusive activities that seniors with joint issues can incorporate into their lives. There are many more to explore based on your physical ability, your location, and ultimately your desire to stay active. Other activities not mentioned but are also considered low impact would be golf, gardening, ballroom or line dancing, elliptical training, and Nordic walking. There are so many things we can do to keep moving and to keep healthy!

Final Tips: Stay hydrated throughout the day, especially before and after your exercises. Include a 5-minute warm-up before and a cool-down after your exercise sessions. Modify the intensity of the exercises to your comfort level. If something hurts, stop doing it. Take breaks as needed during exercise, especially if you feel pain or discomfort. And most importantly, choose activities that you enjoy, as this will help you stay consistent with any exercise plan!

If you found this book helpful, if it provided you with a foundation to get active in spite of a health issue, I would greatly appreciate it if you could leave a favorable review for the book on Amazon so others can find it too!

8

Resources

Burkam, M.D.,B (2024). *Your aching joints: Normal aging or something else?*. Summa Health. https://www.summahealth.org/medicalservices/seniors/timely-tips/normal-aging-and-wellness/your-aching-joints

CDC Staff(2019, October 18). *Fit & Strong! program description.* Centers for Disease Control and Prevention. https://www.cdc.gov/arthritis/interventions/programs/fit-strong.htm

Cleveland Clinic Medical Professionals. (2023, November 13). *What is the main cause of arthritis?*. Cleveland Clinic. https://my.clevelandclinic.org/health/diseases/12061-arthritis

Haskins, J. (2018, September 1). *Living healthier through low-impact exercise.* The Nation's Health. https://www.thenationshealth.org/content/48/7/16

Dr. Lam, P., & Miller, M. (2015, April 17). *Why Tai Chi for arthritis?*. Tai Chi for Health Institute. https://taichiforhealthinstitute.org/why-tai-chi-for-arthritis/

Mayo Clinic Staff (2023, August 29). *Arthritis*. Mayo Clinic https://w
ww.mayoclinic.org/diseases-conditions/arthritis/symptoms-causes/
syc-20350772

Sears, B. (2022, February 22). *Looking for a minimal stress workout? try
low-impact exercise*. Verywell Health. https://www.verywellhealth.com
/low-impact-exercise-5216089